MORNING & EVENING YOGA

JANITA STENHOUSE

POLAIR PUBLISHING
LONDON

First published April 2006

Text and Drawings © Janita Stenhouse, 2006

British Library Cataloguing-in-Publication Data
A catalogue record for this book is available from the British Library

ISBN 1-905398-09-3

Set in Palladio at the Publishers
Printed and bound in Great Britain by Cambridge University Press

CONTENTS

Acknowledgments

My grateful thanks are due to:
Fabien Cimetière for the beautiful photography
Jane Stenhouse and Philippe Fradin for modelling for the photos
Terri Hilder and Michael "Scotty" Kane for modelling for the drawings
Alma Stenhouse for all her help and encouragement
Colum Hayward for his sensitive editing
Dr Ananda Balayogi Bhavanani for his help with the mantras
And last but by no means least, my teachers for their inspiration :
Lakshmi Waters, Dr. Swami Gitananda Giri,
Dr Swami Anandakapila Saraśwati, and B.K.S. Iyengar.

Om shanthi.

CHAPTER ONE : LARKS AND OWLS

YOU SET off for your regular yoga class feeling tired, stressed, with maybe an incipient headache. You're not at your best. After an hour and a half, possibly two hours of stretching, conscious breathing, relaxation and maybe meditation, you come out feeling great, totally relaxed and tranquil. You wish you could always feel this way.

Your teacher tells you that yoga is something you can do every day, but you find a hundred reasons (often really creative ones!) for not being able to find the time to spend an hour and a half at home doing yoga. But why be so hard on yourself? Why insist on a full session that would mean setting aside a large chunk of your day, when you can get the same amount of benefit from doing one or two much shorter sessions? You would even be better off doing a daily short session than one long session once or twice a week. Your body actually prefers regular short sessions, and will attain and then retain its suppleness much better this way. And there's another very good reason for practising regularly: you can help yourself to get much more out of your waking hours by optimizing your body functions and doing one or two short sessions per day.

So you check out the poses in your yoga manual and find scores, maybe even hundreds of poses. You are faced with the dilemma of multiple choice! So instead of confusing you with a plethora of poses from which to choose for your daily short sessions, this book proposes two sequences, each containing all the elements of a traditional yoga class. You'll also find suggestions for enhancing your practice with energy-centre (*chakra*) consciousness and with *mantra*-chanting, and you'll find a glossary at the back explaining the Sanskrit terms (anything in italics in the text). And the reason I have chosen these two particular sequences is that they address two kinds of people: the larks and the owls.

Are you up with the lark, or are you a night-owl? Do you wake before the alarm has a chance to ring, or

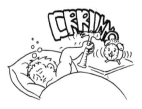

do you reach groggily for the snooze button when the thing finally goes off (too darn soon!)?

By nine o'clock, is your evening just beginning; or are you already looking forward to bed? Only thirty per cent of people fall into the two extremes, but the other seventy per cent do have tendencies toward one end of the scale or the other. And these tendencies are often affected by our job, whether we have small children, what age we are, or whether we are in good health.

Whether we are larks or owls, we probably wish we could feel like a lark in the mornings, and keep going like an owl in the evenings—especially if we live with someone of the opposite tendency. But how do you do this without exhausting yourself? There's a simple answer: reset your biological clock.

The biological clock

There exists in the centre of your brain a tiny pea-sized gland called the pineal gland—simply because it looks rather like a tiny pine cone. At birth it can weigh up to forty grams, but it begins to atrophy after we reach twelve years old, and with age tends also to calcify (Swami Anandakapila Saraśwati likes to joke that we really do have rocks in our heads!). This pineal gland is your biological clock, controlling many natural body-cycles such as your sleep-cycle, body-temperature, blood-hormone levels, blood-pressure, how alert you are and your susceptibility to disease. When you are in good health, your body-rhythms work in synchronicity, like a finely-tuned orchestra. The pineal gland is photosensitive, and is literally a 'third eye', the *ajna chakra* of yoga. As night falls and light-levels diminish, it increases its production of melatonin, and as day dawns it reduces production. In fact, night-time levels of melatonin are usually ten times what they are in daylight hours. Interestingly meditation, relaxation and visualization also enhance its production.

Melatonin is also produced in the retina of the eyes and in the gut but mainly in the pineal gland. Production is high in infancy and lessens as we get older, and this may be why we sleep less at eighty than we did at the age of eight. It regulates the production of growth hormones and the onset of puberty and of menopause, strengthens the immune system, and being antioxidant it is very effective as a free radical scavenger (better even than Vitamins C and E which can't easily cross the blood–brain barrier); it may even affect the production of tumours, as low melatonin levels have been detected in patients suffering from cancer. Melatonin levels are also low in people suffering from Seasonal Affective Disorder, from jetlag, heart disease, sleep disorders and in children with Attention Deficit Hyperactivity Disorder.

However, exposure to light reduces production. If we are constantly exposed to light, whether natural or artificial, we are lowering our melatonin production. This is why travelling across timezones and working night shifts have such a powerful negative effect on our sleep-patterns and our general health.

During the day, the pineal gland organizes the production of another hormone, serotonin. It regulates mood, emotions, appetite, pain-perception, blood pressure, and memory. Low serotonin levels are common in people who are suffering from depression or are suicidal. The pineal gland processes both melatonin and serotonin from tryptophan, which occurs in meat, fish, chocolate, oats, bananas, dried dates, milk, cottage cheese and peanuts. (This is not a good excuse to eat nothing but chocolate and peanuts of course!)

It is only quite recently that western science has discovered much about this gland and research is ongoing. But amazingly, the yogis of ancient India who may not have studied at the local Faculty of Medicine nevertheless certainly knew their physiology and anatomy, and appreciated that sunlight stimulates the pineal gland and regulates its production of hormones, and thus its importance on the rest of the organism, and on whether you are a night-owl or an early bird. They also worked out that disrupting the circadian rhythm leads to ill-health.

But what exactly decides how your personal body-clock works? Obviously the body will respond to light and dark, but even if you spend days in total darkness your body tends to remain on a twenty-four- to twenty-five-hour cycle (hence the name circadian—*circa diem*, Latin for 'about a day'). Genes also have a part to play here, and there's even a theory that we are genetically programmed to have different circadian rhythms so that back in the dawn of humankind, there would always be someone awake to tend the fires and make sure no animals or hostile clans invaded the cave while everyone else was asleep. (I would hope we've evolved a bit since then…)

So if your body is unwilling to get going at the crack of dawn, when your boss is expecting you to be ultra-efficient and fully alert, what can you do? And what to do when you have just travelled halfway round the world and need to be on the ball to give a talk to a prestigious audience?

Most adults need between seven and nine hours of sleep and if your reflex on hearing the alarm is to hit the snooze button, the best thing you can do for your body is to go to bed earlier. Another way is to get up at a regular time and practise yoga to re-programme your metabolism so that getting up is no longer a challenge. I suggest you try practising *sûrya namaskâr*, the 'Salutation to the Sun', every morning when you get up—research shows that people who exercise in the mornings sleep better and find making fitness a regular habit much easier than those who exercise in the evening. Another reason to practise *sûrya namaskâr* is that it is a regular sequence of movements, so you don't have to think 'what'll I do next?'.

And in order to remain fresh and alert as evening arrives, try practising *chandra namaskâr*, the 'Salute to the Moon', in the late afternoon or early evening. Both these sequences come to us from *hatha yoga* and combine postures that move the body in several ways to stretch and tone the whole organism. And each sequence takes only a few minutes to practise. Because you practise at your own rhythm and then pass a pleasant few minutes relaxing and concentrating on your breathing, you are not left panting and exhausted afterwards

but relaxed and energized. The short period of relaxation or meditation at the end allows the body to assimilate the benefits and dissolve any lactic acid that may have built up in the muscles.

Are you a lark or an owl?

Larks tend to wake early and have no need for an alarm clock, and even on holiday they have a tendency to wake up at about the same time as on a workday. Their favourite meal may well be breakfast! These are not morning grouches and don't need a huge caffeine boost to start their day. They are at their best before noon and by evening are beginning to run out of steam. Night-shift work is not recommended for larks, and they suffer more from jetlag than do owls. They fall asleep faster than owls and go to bed earlier, so their peak melatonin secretion period is about 3.30 am—for owls the peak melatonin secretion period is two hours later.

Owls find morning a difficult time of day! They really need at least one alarm clock but several are better, and they often skip breakfast altogether. They tend to be late arrivals at work and will get up late on holiday and at weekends because they can. Their caffeine intake is often much higher than larks', and quite honestly their mood in the morning can only be described as bearish! On the plus side, owls adapt faster than larks to change of timezones so suffer less from jetlag and cope better with shift work. They take longer to fall asleep, but during the daytime they fall asleep more easily than larks—a siesta for owls is a pleasure. The problem for owls living in hot countries is that they miss out on the cool morning freshness, whereas larks have trouble keeping going in the evening when things start to happen! For example, in India the streets come alive with market stalls in the evening, and the Spanish consider 10 pm rather early for dining.

We are not really programmed to function best at night. The evidence: we can't see in the dark. But as many as twenty per cent of the population are more alert in the evening than in the morning. This is particularly true of the fifteen- to twenty-five age-group, regardless of the genetic set-up, owing to surges in reproductive hormones that affect the production of melatonin and create a 'temporary owl phase'. Only about ten per cent of the population find that morning is their optimum time and by 9 pm are more or less ready for bed. This group includes a lot of over-sixties, and parents of very young children.

However most people fall between these two extremes, having only lark or owl tendencies. Which category do you fit most? Which part of the day do you usually feel at your best? And would you like to be able to wake up feeling alert and ready for anything, but also be able to keep going through the evening and enjoy evening activities? These things are possible if you learn to reset your body clock. One of the most efficient ways of resetting your body clock is to practise yoga first thing in the morning, even briefly, and again in the early evening. Yoga has bequeathed to us two sequences that are tailored to do just this; they are *sûrya namaskâr*, the Salutation to the Sun, and *chandra namaskâr*, the Salutation to the Moon.

Tips for coping for larks

To stay bright-eyed and full of energy in the evening is hard for a lark, so in the early evening practise *chandra namaskâr* or take a walk in the fresh air, to help you stay fresh longer and put off that ready-for-bed feeling.

Make sure that there's plenty of light in the evening—low lighting may be relaxing and romantic but your eyes will start to droop sooner.

You wake up at 3 am and can't get back to sleep? This is an hour that is often a tricky moment of the night. Larks' lowest heart rate is about 3 am (for owls it's at its lowest over three hours later), and according to the Chinese this is the moment in the twenty-four hour cycle when the liver energy, which was in the ascendant since 1am, hands over to lung energy for two hours.

If you do wake at 3 am and can't get back to sleep, don't fight it but try rhythmic breathing (see the section on relaxation). This will distract your brain and allow it to relax. If you were woken by your bladder and you have to go to the toilet, don't put on any bright lights, and have a low wattage bulb in the bathroom. Close your bedroom curtains every night, especially around full moon, to keep light levels low.

Tips for coping for owls

To help reset your body clock, try to get up at the same time every day, even on holiday, even if you went to bed late! You can always take a short nap in the afternoon to catch up on lost sleep, and twenty minutes in the afternoon is better than a longer nap as you won't wake up feeling groggy. Every morning, do *sûrya namaskâr* as soon as you can after waking, in order to stimulate your metabolism. It does this better than a pot of coffee and the side-effects are far more beneficial.

A morning routine helps you to function smoothly without having to think about what you have to do. This is why *sûrya namaskâr* is a good sequence to do—the movements become more fluid with practice and the body knows what comes next. The help this muscle-memory brings is a real boon for owls, who are not at their best at this time of the day. Exposure to daylight in the morning can make you more alert earlier in the day.

In the evening don't watch television or exercise late; read or listen to music instead. Leave the bedroom curtains open so that the morning light wakes you gently and gradually, which is so much more pleasant and kinder to the nerves than a shrill alarm.

Whether you are a lark or an owl, remember that you are capable of teaching yourself new skills. The skill of resetting your body clock is one of them. If you can learn to play tennis, or write with your other hand, or lose weight, you can teach your body to get up and function well in the morning, and to stay alert and function well in the evening! And if you are a lark living with an owl, or vice versa, resetting your body clock can make life a lot more harmonious and help you synchronise with each other.

When you wake up, roll over on your left side for a few minutes to activate your right nostril and stimulate the left hemisphere of your brain. Then spend a while stretching luxuriously like a cat so that you wake your body up gently but effectually. Try not to swallow your saliva yet, but head for the bathroom and rinse your mouth thoroughly—notice how already you're feeling fresher. If you have a tongue scraper, use it, or else use the edge of a spoon to scrape any gunk off your tongue, from as far back as possible. The tongue spends the night collecting toxins and acids, and you don't want to reabsorb all that! Cleaning your tongue will not only remove toxins but ensure your breath is sweet.

Why do yoga in the morning?

The word 'yoga' comes from the Sanskrit root *yug* meaning a yoke. Yoga, by yoking and controlling the energies latent in the complex being that is You, works to unite and balance the physical, the mental/emotional, and the spiritual parts of you, to make a strong and unified whole. Yoga's aim is to establish that unity to show you your true Self, the unchanging and true You. As human beings, we tend to hide behind façades of personality and habits accrued over the years. We genuinely believe that this confusion of habits and mannerisms is our true Self and we can go through life without being disabused of this illusion. Occasionally due to good luck or unusual circumstances we might glimpse the true Self tucked away behind all that, but rarely and rather inconsistently. Yoga renews our contacts with our Self. The balancing and gently penetrating method of yoga works so effectively because it works from the inside. You can work at your own pace, to your own personal needs, respecting your day-to-day changes.

Yoga developed in Northern India several thousand years ago, in a culture so removed in every sense from our twenty-first century western culture that you may wonder how it could be of genuine help. In fact yoga fits ideally into our busy modern lifestyle because it demands very little but gives you a great deal in return. The fast pace of modern life leaves us feeling we have no time for ourselves.

So often I hear people say 'I'd like to do yoga but I can't find the time.' To find time every day for a full classical yoga session is difficult, especially if you have a heavy workload, lots of responsibilities and a busy social life, but practising these two sequences requires only five or ten minutes, twice a day. While they aren't quite the same as a full yoga session, the sequences nevertheless contain the elements of *âsana* (posture), *prânâyâma* (breath control) and *dhâranâ* (concentration) essential to such a session, while taking only a fraction of the time.

The physical, mental/emotional and spiritual benefits that accrue from performing *sûrya namaskâr* for between five and ten minutes in the morning and *chandra namaskâr* for a few minutes in the evening will quickly become apparent and in only a short time you'll wonder how you could afford not to practise some yoga daily. The benefits outlined below may seem extravagant at first, but with less than a month's practice you'll be able to feel and see the difference that yoga makes to your life.

'Woke up this morning….'

How you start your day affects how you live the rest of it—remember the old saying 'got out of bed on the wrong side'? *Sûrya namaskâr* makes you feel you've gotten out of the right side of the bed, by creating a positive attitude that gives you a good foundation for the rest of the day.

So what is *sûrya namaskâr* ? It is a sequence of movements found in *hatha yoga* which is practised rhythmically, accompanied by full, deep breathing and often by *mantras*. There are many forms of this sequence, varying in length and difficulty. Some forms have as few as four positions, while others have up to thirty-three movements. The version detailed here contains postures that move your body in all the ways that are possible—forward, backward, sideways, twisting, and inverted, accompanied by rhythmic breathing and concentration—in fact, all the elements of a full yoga session, so it is perfect for early morning practice. The best-known version, the Rishikesh *sûrya namaskâr*, lacks the lateral stretches and the twists included here. *Sûrya namaskâr* can take about five minutes or a quarter of an hour, depending on your personal needs and speed. It has profoundly beneficial physical and mental effects so that, practised first thing in the morning, it improves not only your health but also your outlook. It is a physical celebration of the transition of night into day, of unconsciousness to consciousness, of the return of one's *manas* from sleep to awareness. It is a physical dedication by the yogi or yogini to be present in the Here and Now. Daily practice brings sunshine into your life irrespective of the weather!

Where are you at this moment?

If you can practise in a garden with a good view of the sun as it rises, you are fortunate. If you are in a sixth-floor apartment with a good view of rain falling on the factory next door, you have a wonderful opportunity to exercise your imagination. And if you are somewhere like Finland, your imagination may have to provide you with a great deal of sunrises. The closer you are to the Equator, the less variation in the time of sunrise.

Clearly an actual sunrise will make your practice easier and more effective, but don't despair if the sun rises at a really inconvenient hour or it's raining where you are. Some people simplify matters by hanging a picture of a sunrise on the wall, but you don't really need this. Your mind can provide you with a beautiful sunrise.

So prepare yourself for your practice, both physically and mentally. Don't succumb to the temptation to have just a bite of breakfast first—it really is much more effective and comfortable to do the sequence on an empty stomach.

If necessary, close your eyes and, on the blackboard behind your eyelids, allow the image of a cloudless night sky to appear. As your breathing deepens and becomes even, let your imaginary sky begin to lighten; and as you come to attention in *samasthiti*, the dawn draws closer. As you place

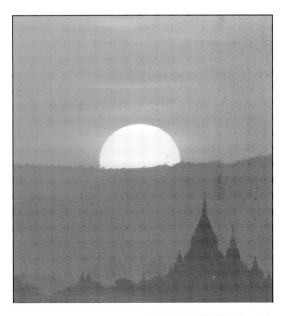

your palms together at your heart centre, the first rays of sunlight appear over the horizon. Keep the mental picture going as you begin your physical practice so that by the end, as you stand once more in *samasthiti*, palms together at *anâhata chakra*, you are bathed in the warm rays of the risen sun.

If you're like me, morning is not your best time of day, and the idea of jumping out of bed and launching into a series of physical jerks is absolute anathema. Fortunately this is something entirely different, so there's nothing to fear. At first the temptation (especially for owls) to snuggle down into the bedcovers may seem insuperable, and even after a couple of days may still seem preferable. But the trick to overcoming sloth is—don't think, just do. I can't actually *promise* that you'll find it easier to get out of bed, but I can assure you that once you establish a good rhythm of practice you'll find the waking-up process much easier. And I speak as an owl who finds this is the case.

To begin with, you may experience some tightness in the tendons (especially in the backs of the legs), stiffness caused by muscular tension and by toxic deposits in the joints, and perhaps a lack of coordination. Please resist the temptation to work through the pain—at best this will only give you extra tightness in the muscles and tendons, and

at worst may even damage them, setting you back several weeks. Never go beyond stretch to pain. By working gently and maintaining the integrity of each movement, and respecting the present (not immutable) state of your body and its capacity, you'll find that as the days pass suppleness, flexibility, coordination and efficient use of muscles develop naturally.

The gunas

According to yoga philosophy, everything in creation is composed of three qualities in various unequal proportions. These three qualities are known as *sattva*—intelligence, purity ; *rajas*—passion, activity ; and *tamas*—inertia, mass.

If you are predominantly *tamas* in the morning,

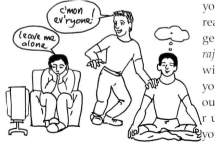

you'll have real trouble getting up. A *rajas* mood will have you leaping out of bed, rushing your practice through, perhaps over-stretching and working up a good sweat. In a *sattvic* mood you are calm and serene throughout, practising with integrity and full of awareness; ideally, this is your aim.

Other considerations

Your attitude affects your practice, of course. When I wake up in the morning I'm normally not quite back in my physical body yet—I'm an owl obliged by life to be a lark. If I have to speak to anybody before doing *sûrya namaskâr*, I sound very different—my voice has a much lower timbre. Usually as I roll out of bed, head for the bathroom and then for my mat and my practice, I haven't really got going mentally at all, I'm on automatic pilot and in fact there's so little going on up top that it's the kind of mind just right for meditation, given a little disciplined concentration. And in fact as the practice evolves, it becomes a meditation in motion. I find that after *sûrya namaskâr*, I am far more ready for whatever the day has in store for me.

Sometimes when you wake up, you've just had a dream and

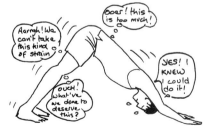

it lingers. This will affect your *sûrya namaskâr*. The kind of sleep you've had affects your *sûrya namaskâr*, too. Of course, whether you're a lark or an owl will affect your *sûrya namaskâr*. But don't let all that put you off ! The mere doing of *sûrya namaskâr* will sort out your mind and leave it refreshed, calm and ready to face whatever the day has to offer with equanimity and fortitude.

It's time I mentioned the necessity for modesty and acceptance. In any yoga class you're told : 'there's no competition in yoga', and you know that this applies equally to competition with yourself. But what I'm trying to say here is that your approach to your practice is best when entirely uncritical. If I begin and find my fingers don't even reach my knees (let alone the floor) in my first *pâdahastâsana*, the ego attempts to make a judgmental remark. Later on in the series as it gets easier to lay the whole hand flat on the floor, again the ego may intervene with some praise to sidetrack my mind altogether. Don't let it! Remember who's in control! Remember the advice given in the *Bhagavad-Gitâ*: 'action for its own sake with no thought of reward'.

Sadly, *sûrya namaskâr* has

been downgraded in certain yoga schools here in the West to a limbering sequence in yoga sessions. But first thing in the morning, stiffened by several hours of relative immobility in a prone position, it's a good idea to limber up a bit before your practice, especially if it's cold. A good shaking-out of the limbs can be sufficient in warm weather, although a spine with problems would appreciate a few gentle twisting and stretching movements. Then start the *sûrya namaskâr* sequence gently, with plenty of attention to ensure the body is comfortable. Take it easy and never over-stretch, especially if the weather is cold and humid. This is another place where you should tailor your practice to your personal needs, which can alter widely from one day to the next.

Both sequences, *sûrya namaskâr* and *chandra namaskâr*, benefit us on many levels. On the physical level, the benefits quickly become apparent as body functions improve. On the mental level, they focus the 'grasshopper mind' and calm it. On the spiritual level, one acknowledges the Creative Force, by whatever name one uses for That. Yoga works to strengthen and balance the three parts of the body—body, mind, soul.

One of my yoga students once asked me if *sûrya namaskâr* might in fact be a form of sun worship, because if so, he felt that as a devout Christian, he could not be a party to it. Don't worry, I told him. The Salute to the Sun is suitable for people of all religions and beliefs, as well as non-believers. It is non-denominational! The sun happens to be the largest manifestation of the Creative Force visible to the naked eye. It is the most important source of energy and life for the planet, and all that exists on it. *Sûrya namaskâr* acknowledges these facts.

You may wonder why I suggest you should get up before dawn for this. Why not do it later in the day when you have more time and are more supple? Quite simply because it is the best time of the day to do it—it is quiet, it is tranquil, nobody else is around to distract you, and the suppleness and calm that ensue set you up so well for the day. It is a time when you can easily tune in to nature and to the spirit within you. Besides, the sun's rays are at their most beneficial at sunrise and sunset (having to pass further through the atmosphere), whereas later in the day they can be quite harmful and destructive even in quite non-tropical latitudes, and especially where there are holes in the ozone layer.

Traditionally, the correct time for *sûrya namaskâr* is during the *brahma muhurta*—that is, between 4 and 6 am, when there is little activity or noise and the earth's energies are neutral (as they are also at sunset). This refers, of course, to sunrise in India, where the length of the days is fairly even. Clearly if you live in a latitude where sunrise varies considerably over the year, a set time is advisable for convenience. And just think how rarely you'd be doing *sûrya namaskâr* if you lived within the Arctic Circle!

So as a compromise, I would suggest you get up just before your usual rising time, giving yourself sufficient time to do your ablutions, and then your practice, followed by relaxation or meditation, without feeling rushed at all.

When *sûrya namaskâr* is performed quickly, it stimulates the active energies in the body, which is excellent for waking you up in the morning. If you are a natural lark or the hyperactive type and don't need to be stimulated first thing in the morning, or you're practising later in the day and need to slow down, then by practising *sûrya namaskâr* slowly with a full breath in each posture, you stimulate the passive energies, leaving you calm and meditative—an excellent remedy for the fast pace of modern life. Another reason for practising slowly is that you can give yourself time in each *âsana* to make adjustments so that the posture is more comfortable and safer—there is protection in perfection.

Words of caution for complete beginners
(quite a good idea to read them anyway!)

When you first start to practise *sûrya* and *chandra namaskâr* daily you'll find that the flow of movement causes the body to cleanse itself—there will be a throwing-off of toxins wherever they have built up, whether in the digestive system, in joints, muscles, or wherever, so remember to start with only a couple of rounds and work up gradually as the days pass. If you attempt six rounds from the start, by the third day you can be sure your muscles will be stiff and sore. You may even find you have a runny nose, diarrhoea or a headache, as your body struggles to rid itself of toxins in a hurry.

By starting with a modest number of rounds and building up gradually, you enable your body to effect its cleansing at a reasonable pace. You may well be using muscles that haven't had a decent stretch for quite a while, so be gentle with them! Give them a chance to wake up gently rather than shocking them—the first precept of yoga is non-violence (for the precepts of yoga see page 55). If you feel pain, this means you are doing it wrong! Pain sends the body into alarm mode, causing the release of adrenalin, the 'fight-or-flight' hormone, and causing the muscles to contract, so there's no longer any possibility of stretching.

If you have coronary heart disease, high blood-pressure, a hernia, intestinal tuberculosis, or have had a stroke, it's probably safer not to practise either *sûrya namaskâr* or *chandra namaskâr*, certainly not without the authorization of your doctor, and trained supervision. If you have slipped disc, sciatica, or had abdominal surgery in the last twelve months, please check with your doctor before embarking on practice.

If you have a detached retina, it is better to avoid any inverted postures, and the same applies to women who are menstruating. If so, avoid *padahastâsana* in *sûrya namaskâr*, and *adho mukha śvânâsana* in both *sûrya* and *chandra namaskâr*. Furthermore, if your periods tend to be very heavy, delay practice for the first two or three days of menstruation. You should check the disclaimer and the note on page 31 if you are pregnant. Whatever the case, always remember to respect the state of your body *as it is today*, and never be tempted to do more than your intuition tells you is right for you at the moment. No competition, no hurry, just living in the present in full consciousness.

Remember that unless you have a real problem with the nose, respiration should always be through the nostrils. It's what they are there for, after all. If you have a cold, then before commencing practice it's a good idea to clear them thoroughly. See the section on breathing below. A good honk on a hanky isn't as good as *jala neti* (see p. 53, and ask your yoga teacher to teach you this).

The breathing throughout both of these practices is smooth and deep. If your breathing becomes jerky, it will affect your balance as well as interrupt the flow of oxygen to the muscles which will quickly tire. A simple rule of thumb for breathing in both of these sequences is: any forward bend or lateral stretch is accompanied by an exhalation; any backward stretch is accompanied by an inhalation. Most twists are done on an exhalation, although they can also be done on inhalation, which will expand the ribcage and protect the dorsal vertebrae from compression.

What you will need for practice

Wear loose and comfortable clothing. Any firm, non-skid surface will do to practice on, and make sure you have enough room to move freely without banging into furniture. Preferably there should be no interruptions (so switch off phones and bells, and put the cat or dog out). Try to avoid practising in a close and stuffy atmosphere.

CHAPTER TWO : SALUTATION TO THE SUN

WE COME now to the actual procedure for *sûrya namaskâr*, beginning with the preparation.

Samasthiti: upright and steady.

Samasthiti is also known as *tadâsana*, the mountain pose. This is the basic standing posture and deserves all the attention accorded to it here!

Stand with the feet hip-width apart and parallel. Lift the toes (to stretch the skin of the soles) and spread them like a fan, then replace them on the mat without tensing them.

Lift the insteps without rolling the feet outwards (imagine an upturned saucer under them) and check that the weight is distributed evenly throughout the feet in two arcs.

The legs are straight without any hyper-extension in the backs of the knees. Lift the hip-bones so the pubis moves towards the navel, and because you are using the abdominals to do this, the coccyx will drop down and forward so that the pelvis tilts backward a little, to lengthen the lower back and redress any tendency to lordosis. (I used to have a terrible lordosis before I began practising yoga regularly.)

Lift the breastbone, widen the collarbones, and lower the shoulderblades towards the waist, to relax the shoulders downwards and away from the ears. Relax the arms completely so they hang comfortably by the sides.

Lengthen the entire spine, feeling each vertebra lift away from the one below. Feel the stretch from the coccyx right up through the crown of the head.

Check the stretch in the nape of the neck—the face should be vertical, the chin level, and from the side the ears are in line with the shoulders, hips and heels (you have to imagine that!).

Spend a few moments relaxing the muscles of the forehead, eyes and jaw, and also relax your tongue—let it float freely in the mouth. Allow this relaxation of the face to accompany you right through the practice.

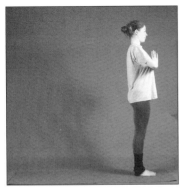
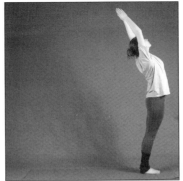
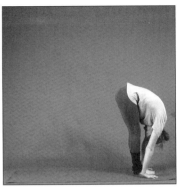

1) Pranâmâsana
—the greeting pose

In *samasthiti*, place the palms together at the heart centre so that the knuckles of the thumbs press lightly on the 'sea of tranquillity' acupressure point midway between the nipples. Observe your breath and let it become long and smooth, as you centre your mind.

2) Hasta uttânâsana
—the upward stretch

As you inhale deeply, stretch the arms up keeping the palms together, and lift and arch the back to open the chest and abdomen. Keep your eyes open to prevent possible dizziness and keep the shoulders relaxed and down by bringing the shoulder blades down and inwards. Feel the stretch from the toes to the fingertips.

If you have back problems, keep the stretch vertical, widen your arms and keep the shoulder blades wide also. You can also bend your knees a little to avoid any pressure in the lower back. If you are pregnant, skip this posture and move straight on to the next.

3) Pâdahastâsana
—the hands-to-feet pose

Exhale as you fold forward from the hips to bring your hands to either side of your feet, trying to keep the back flat—keep the front of the spine extended and relax the muscles of the back. Tighten the perineum, or more precisely the anterior sphincter (*mûla*

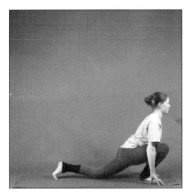 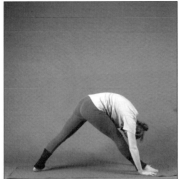 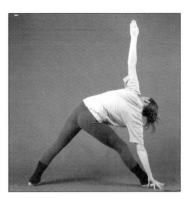

bandha). If your hands don't arrive on the mat at either side of the feet, bend the knees.

4) Aśwa sanchalanâsana —the horseman pose

Inhaling, release *mûla bandha* and step back with the left leg, placing the knee on the floor. Bring the hips forward as if to sit on the right heel, open your chest, relax your shoulders and face, lengthen the back of the neck so that in looking up you don't compress the cervical

spine. Try to keep the skin and muscles of the thighs soft and allow the hamstrings to lengthen. If your cervical vertebrae are fragile, keep the face vertical. If knee injury makes sitting forward towards the heel unwise, keep the shin vertical.

5) Pârśvottânâsana —the forward stretch pose

Exhaling (*mûla bandha*), straighten the right leg, and if you are supple keep the body in contact with the thigh. Press

down a little with the outer edge of the right foot and with the left big toe to keep the insteps lifted and the legs active. Check that the weight is evenly distributed between the two feet. Feel the rotation of the thighs outward to open the hips. Relax the shoulders, ribcage, back, arms— and face.

6) Trikonâsana —the triangle pose

Inhaling, turn the torso to the left, lift the left hand up to vertical and turn the head gently to look at the palm of the left hand—no sudden movements of the head! Keep the neck long and relaxed, open the chest by stretching the two hands apart, and ensure the right side of the ribcage is extended so that the right ribs are not compressed. This is easier if the right hand is lifted onto the fingertips. Don't allow your head to drop down out of alignment with the spine.

Usually one exhales to go into *trikonâsana*, but by inhaling into it, the ribcage is expanded and the spinal vertebrae are protected.

7)
Exhale (*mûla bandha*) as you return the left hand to the floor beside the right foot into *pârśvottânâsana*. Ease the body along the thigh and relax the back and shoulders. A smile will always relax both the face and the mind (and release

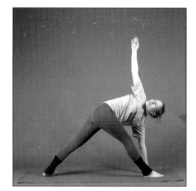 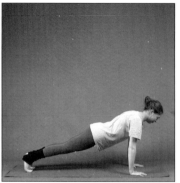

endorphins, those delightful feel-good hormones, into the brain).

8) Parivrrta trikonâsana —the reversed triangle pose
Inhale as you turn the torso to the right, lift the right hand to vertical and turn the head gently to look at the right palm. As in *trikonâsana*, keep the spine long on both sides, and open the chest by extending the hands away from each other. Here too, press down with the outer edge of the right foot and the left big toe as before.

9)
Exhale as you bring the right hand to the floor beside the foot to return to *pârśvottânâsana*. (*mûla bandha*) keeping the legs active and relaxing the shoulders, back, arms and face.

10) Santolanâsana —the plank pose
Inhale as you step the right foot back beside the left foot, lifting up onto the toes, then bringing the body into a smooth and even diagonal line.

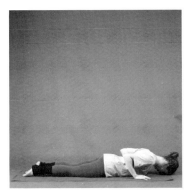 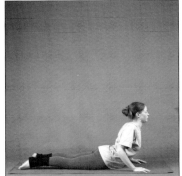 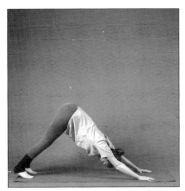

11) Bhujangâsana —the cobra pose

Bend the elbows and knees, and bring the lower half of the body to the ground, the upper part of the body supported by the arms, keeping the shoulders down and the elbows close to the ribs. Open the chest using a downward and inward movement of the shoulder blades, keep the nape of the neck long, and let the face remain vertical—a cobra stares straight ahead in order to hypnotise its prey. Lengthen the tailbone down towards the mat to protect the lumbar spine.

Classically, this posture is done with breath-retention (*kumbhaka*), though you should breathe normally if you need to.

12) Adho mukha śvânâsana —the downward-facing dog pose

Exhale as you lift the hips high, letting the heels drop towards the mat, and feel the delicious stretch along the entire spine and the backs of the legs. Lift the shoulders away from the wrists and relax the neck completely. Let the head sink between the arms towards the floor. Check that the pressure on the palms of the hands is distributed evenly by pressing a little with base of the thumbs.

This is a superb stretch for tight hamstrings and the popliteal tendons behind the knees so if your knees tend to over-extend, gently lift the quadriceps muscles in the thighs to lift the kneecaps and protect the knees.

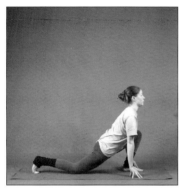 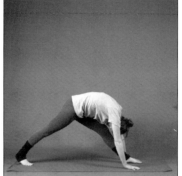 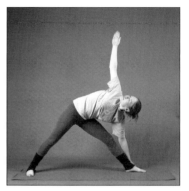

13) Aśwa sanchalanâsana —the horseman pose

Inhale as you swing the left leg forward to place the foot between the hands. Bring the hips forward and down, open the chest, draw the shoulderblades down, lengthen the spine and look up if your cervical vertebrae will allow it, maintaining the length in the back of the neck to prevent any compression of the carotid artery or pressure on the vertebrae. Here too it may be easier to place the hands on the tips of the fingers rather than keep the palms flat on the floor.

If the foot doesn't arrive between the hands (and this is possibly the hardest part of the sequence) you have two options: grab the ankle and lift the foot forward, or slide the rest of your body back to join the foot! This latter does tend to make you end up rather further back than you started out so make sure there's room behind you.

14) Pârśvottânâsana—the forward stretch pose

Exhaling, straighten the left leg, hopefully keeping the body to the thigh. Don't panic if this is not possible yet (*mûla bandha*).

15) Trikonâsana —the triangle pose

Inhaling, turn the torso to the left, lift the left hand up to vertical and turn the head gently towards the palm of the left hand. Keep the neck long and relaxed, open the chest by stretching the two hands apart,

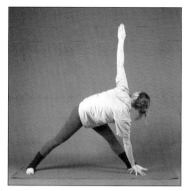

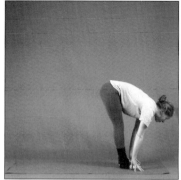

and ensure the right-hand side ribs are extended so that the right side is not compressed.

16)
Exhale as you return the left hand to the floor beside the right foot into *pârśvottânâsana* and relax the whole spine (*mûla bandha*).

(17) Parivrrta trikonâsana —the reversed triangle pose
Inhale as you turn the torso to the right, lift the right hand to vertical and turn the head to look

at the right palm. Again, keep the spine long on both sides, the head aligned with the spine, and open the chest by extending the hands away from each other.

18)
Exhale as you return the left hand to the floor beside the right foot into *pârśvottânâsana* (*mûla bandha*).

19) Konâsana —the angle pose
Inhale as you bring the right

foot forward to join the left foot between the hands, lifting your head, flattening and lengthening the whole spine. Draw the shoulderblades together and down towards the waist to open the chest and relax the shoulders. Straighten the legs….

20) Pâda hastâsana —the hands-to-feet pose
… and then, exhaling, bring your body towards your thighs and relax the neck completely, allowing the whole spine and head to hang from the hip girdle (*mûla bandha*). Keep the front of the spine extended to protect the spinal vertebrae. Since the invention of chairs, human spines have become weakened so that discs may slip or become damaged. Notice how chairs tend to discourage good sitting posture, especially couches and sofas!

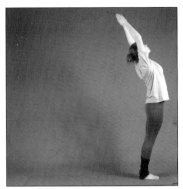

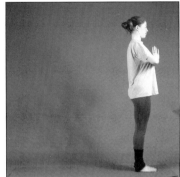

21) Hasta uttânâsana —the upward stretch

As you inhale deeply, open the arms to the sides and then up to vertical; stretch your whole body upwards, and if your back will allow it lean back to open the chest and abdomen. Bringing the arms up at the sides is a lot easier on the back than lifting them up directly in front, and if you have back problems, bend the knees as well. If you are pregnant, simply unroll gently to vertical, keeping the arms relaxed.

(22) Pranâmâsana —the greeting pose

As you exhale, return the hands to the greeting pose at the heart centre, and relax. Observe your breath, then the state of your body and of your mind. How wonderful it is that your body can do this!

Now you have a choice. You can either exhale as you fold forward to repeat all the above postures, leading this time with the right leg to complete the round, or you can stay for a moment in *pranâmâsana*, in an attitude of gratitude. This may form a rest before you start again, observing the effects and reactions, or you may move on to relaxation or meditation.

CHAPTER THREE: AFTER THE NAMASKÂR

SO, YOU'VE done your rounds of *sûrya namaskâr*—what next? Well, this depends on several things, including your location, your metabolism, your timetable, and your plans for the rest of the day.

As to your metabolism, you may feel that a shower is needed to wash away the toxins you've excreted through the skin, but please wait awhile, about half an hour is usual, in order not to dissipate the *prâna* liberated by the practice. Many yogis rub their bodies with their hands after yoga to rub *prâna* into the skin. Furthermore, showering after exercise slows the metabolic rate, as does eating. If you are underweight, this is fine, and showering or bathing, and eating straight after exercise will prevent weight loss. If you wish to lose weight or to maintain your weight, wait awhile, preferably from a half to one hour.

If you've done twelve fast rounds, you'll want to rest in *śavâsana* for awhile. If your rounds were smooth and refreshing, you may wish to sit awhile in meditation. I find that either sitting or lying, practising alternate nostril breathing, really relaxes both the physical body and the mind. If you are outside and it's warm, remember that full sun is not the place for this. If it's not warm, wrap up well—a blanket is always useful. You may feel that you need to cool down but this should happen gradually in order to avoid chilling; your body will lose some heat during relaxation or meditation anyway, so it's a good idea to cover your body.

As you can see, this will affect your timetable. Allow yourself enough time to enjoy your practice, and your meditation or relaxation, then do those things that need to be done—feed the children or animals, walk the dog, go to work or whatever.

Sûrya namaskâr stimulates the sympathetic nervous system. Relaxation following *sûrya namaskâr* allows the parasympathetic nervous system to operate, returning the body to a balanced state as well as releasing tension from the muscles and giving the body time to adjust. During relaxation, the lactic acid that may have built up in the muscles from exercise is washed away. Yoga as a whole, along with relaxation and meditation, is being used by more and more medical specialists as therapy for arteriosclerotic heart disease and to prevent future cardiac deterioration.

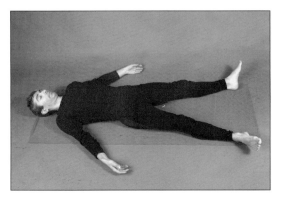

Śavâsana
—the corpse pose

Having finished your rounds, stand erect in *samasthiti* and take several deep, smooth breaths, before lying down and covering yourself with a blanket or light cloth depending on the weather, to retain your energy and warmth. Your feet should be about 45 cm (18 inches) apart and your hands about 25 cm (10 inches) from your hips with the palms up (to relax the upper arms and open your upper chest). Lengthen your spine along the ground by tucking in the chin and tilting the pelvis, then release. If you have lumbar problems, slip a cushion under your thighs; if it's the cervical area that is a problem, slip a cushion under your neck.

Exhale as you close your eyes and make any adjustments necessary to feel comfortable. Be aware of your body—check that the right and left sides are lying equally. Feel your weight being gently given up to gravity to support. Allow your legs to become heavy, then your hips, shoulders, arms, head.

Take three or four deep breaths—inhale through the nose, be aware of the breath in the lungs, then sigh it all out through the mouth, releasing any physical and mental tension along with the breath. Let go.

Take your awareness for a jaunt through your whole body, relaxing each part as you visit it mentally. Let each part soften, broaden, lengthen; let it spread a little. Begin with your feet, move up through the ankles, lower legs, knees, thighs, buttocks, hips, abdomen, along the spine, upper back, ribcage, hands, wrists, lower arms, elbows, upper arms, shoulders, neck, scalp, ears, forehead, eyes, cheeks, nostrils, jaw, lips, tongue, throat.

Your whole body is relaxing, feeling as limp and lifeless as a corpse (hence the name *śavâsana*, the corpse posture) although the mind is still fully alert. Now be aware of your breath and simply watch it as it enters and leaves the body, passing the tips of the nostrils. Feel that, as you inhale, you breathe in peace; as you exhale, you release anything that might prevent total relaxation, physical, mental, emotional. Let go.

Notice how your breathing and heartbeat begin gradually to slow, without you having to do anything about it. Now feel as if you are inhaling only through the left nostril, aiming for the space between your eyebrows, and pause a little before exhaling down the right nostril. Then inhale up the right nostril aiming again for the space between the eyebrows, and after a short pause exhale down the left nostril. At first, the breathing may be a little chaotic, depending on the dynamism of your practice, but gradually you'll be able to install a rhythm; if possible, use *savitrî prânâyâma*, the 2:1 rhythm. Inhale for a count of four, pause for two counts, then exhale for a count of four and rest with lungs empty for a count of two. Gradually lengthen the rhythm to 6:3 or even 8:4 when it feels comfortable, remembering that you never force your breathing. Soon the rhythm becomes automatic and your mind relaxes along with your body. If you find

your mind insists on gadding about, gently return your awareness to your breathing.

When you have relaxed sufficiently, at least for several minutes, release the concentration on the breath and become aware of your whole body. Then gently begin to bring your body back to movement by starting to wriggle your toes and fingers, stretching, yawning and then rolling onto your left side for a moment before sitting up.

Relaxation is a state in which there is no movement, no effort, and the brain becomes quiet—unlike sleep, which includes periods of dreaming during which there is often an increase in muscular tension and the brain is active. In fact deep relaxation can be much more refreshing than sleep.

Meditation

Alternatively, you may prefer to sit for meditation. Choose a comfortable position, one that will allow your whole spine (remember your neck is part of your spine) to be erect, and the chest open, the shoulders relaxed. Not everyone finds the traditional meditation posture *padmâsana*, the Lotus, comfortable, or even possible, though it's to be preferred because of the

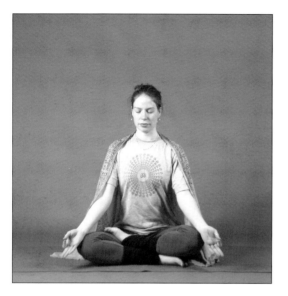

horizontal plane and lengthening your waist. Release any tension in your face and let your shoulders drop away from your ears. Rotate your awareness around your body, as described for *śavâsana*, and settle on your breathing. At first merely observe your respiration, notice its natural rhythm without criticism, without altering it. Then begin *savitrî prânâyâma* as described above: it's much easier to focus the mind on something than on nothing.

If your mind wanders off, gently bring it back to your breathing. Start again. You needn't force it, because the wandering is just a habit it has acquired and with gentle training, will relinquish. When this practice becomes easy, you can begin to focus the mind on itself, watching your thoughts as a passive witness, remaining unattached, until the thoughts become fewer and fewer … until there is peace.

stability it gives. The Half Lotus, *ardha padmâsana,* is also good, but cross-legged will serve, and strictly speaking it is essential only to find a position that keeps your spine erect without outside support and without causing your body to intervene after a while to distract you from your meditation.

Start by relaxing your body once you have it in a good upright posture. Lengthen the spine a little more by slightly drawing your chin back on the

How to adapt the sequence to your personal needs

What I described in the last chapter is a version of the famous Salutation to the Sun, *sûrya namaskâr,* and is fine for most people. However there are some postures in it that you may find difficult or even impossible at present for some reason.

You may have back problems that don't allow you to place your stomach on your thighs in *pâdahastâsana*, in which case flex your knees, especially when coming back up to vertical at the end. Always swing the arms up sideways rather than forwards when returning to vertical to protect the lower back. Concentrate on keeping as much space as possible between the vertebrae—you may find that visualizing the sunshine seeping between them helpful.

In pregnancy, keep the feet well apart, avoid the upward stretches and never stretch too fiercely. Remember that for these nine or ten months you are sharing your body, so treat it with extra respect. In India women are advised to quit the physical practice of *sûrya namaskâr* after the seventh month and to squat and recite the *mantra*s aloud instead. Squatting is excellent for the perineal muscles and the hips, and chanting brings all the benefits of *mantra yoga* to both you and your baby. However, in the western world, most yoga associations are not prepared to recommend this sequence beyond a much earlier stage, and certainly not once the first trimester is coming to an end (12–14 weeks). After the birth you can resume practice when you feel ready, usually after about three months. Take your time getting back to your usual quota of rounds,

let your general energy-level dictate when.

Sometimes you might want to add a little something to pep you up: try adding *mukha bhastrikâ* in the downward-facing dog pose (avoid this altogether if you have a lower-back problem or are pregnant). This respiration is excellent for toning the abdominal muscles and getting the digestive tract going. Inhale through the nose, then purse the lips into an 'O' shape and blast the breath out with force, making a 'whoo' sound. Repeat this breath up to six times, keeping the perineum tightened in *mûla bandha*; the abdominal wall will flap in and out as you breathe because it relaxes outward on the inhalation, and is drawn in brusquely by the exhalation.

When practice becomes smooth and fluid, the sequence gradually becomes imprinted on your muscles and your brain, the breath falls easily into the flow, and your concentration rests easily on what you are doing so that you feel you are truly in your body at this moment (Here and Now), you may want to extend your practice. By concentrating on the energy centres along the spine (see the Glossary under *chakra*) and the movement of *prâna* (bio-energy) within you, you deepen your awareness and enhance the meditational aspect of *sûrya namaskâr*.

The chakras and sûrya namaskâr

The *chakra*s are the centres of subtle energy within the body whose job is to receive the energy flowing in the *nâdîs* and distribute it among the various layers of your Being. These layers include the physical body—see the Glossary under *kośa*. There are many *chakra*s in the body but the best known and most important are all stimulated during this sequence—except *mûladhâra chakra*, the root *chakra*, because it is the seat of *kundalinî*, your cosmic energy. This energy is often called the Serpent Power because it's symbolized as a coiled snake asleep at the base of *suṣumnâ nâdî*, the principal energy channel which runs from the root *chakra* to the top of the head. In activating the other *chakra*s you prepare them for the awakening of *kundalinî*. To disturb this power before your whole system is ready and you are fully mentally prepared can be psychically dangerous—as many western mental institutions can affirm. So, in stimulating all the other *chakra*s except *mûladhâra chakra,* you are as it were preparing the ground without opening the gates.

The *chakra*s are so called because they are wheels or vortices of energy. In Sanskrit, *chakra* means a wheel. Another symbol is a lotus flower. Each centre is a dormant area that, when activated, opens up—like a flower blooming. These centres are located not so much in the physical body as in the subtle body, connecting with the physical body at nerve plexi (see the Glossary for descriptions).

In *sûrya namaskâr* you rotate your awareness through the *chakra*s in coordination with the *âsana*s thus:

pranâmâsana:
anâhata chakra—the heart centre.

hasta uttânâsana:
viśuddha chakra—the throat centre.

pada hastâsana:
svâdhiṣthâna chakra—the pelvic centre.

aśva sanchalanâsana:
ajna chakra—the brow centre or 'third eye'.

pârśvottânâsana:
manipura chakra—the navel centre.

trikonâsana:
manipura chakra—the navel centre.

parivrrta trikonâsana:
manipura chakra—the navel centre.

adho mukha śvânâsana:
viśuddha chakra—the throat centre

bhujangâsana:
svâdhiṣthâna chakra—the pelvic centre.

At first, you may need to spend some time in each *âsana* to get the feel of the *chakra*, but as you become used to locating and visualizing them, and directing your energy there, you'll find your practice speeds up of its own accord. Even though you're working with boosting energy in this mode, please don't be tempted to work too hard and thereby deplete your stamina. The Latin adage *festina lente* applies here: make haste slowly!

The benefits of daily practice

How well do we each know our own body? The vast majority of people seem to consider their bodies as some kind of machinery that can be taken to the doctor when not functioning properly, and the doctor will mend it with weirdly-named and pretty-coloured pills or syrups. How few of us are prepared to take responsibility for the maintenance of this body—which is, after all, the only one we have to live in for the whole of our lives! And it doesn't really take much effort to maintain once in good running order: a few minutes spent exercising the body followed by another few minutes exercising the brain, and you tune the whole organism for the day.

The benefits that accrue from regular practice of this sequence are really impressive and you have only to try it yourself for a few weeks to be convinced of its worth.

The stretching and contraction throughout the sequence wake up muscles, improving blood and lymph circulation, and also your respiration. The controlled rhythmic breathing develops the lungs and the way you use them, boosting oxygen intake which in turn improves the quality of your blood. This freshly-oxygenated blood is circulated throughout the body, nourishing every part, improving the functioning of the internal organs and the condition and quality of your skin. Living in the polluted air of cities often results in poor skin, but yoga offers rejuvenation of the skin tissue, rendering it more elastic and resilient. You may even find that cuts and grazes heal faster. The falling and greying of hair is retarded, as hair and nail cells are revitalised and growth is promoted.

General posture is improved, owing to the

strengthening and development of the muscular and skeletal systems, and stronger bones means less susceptibility to the bone disorders that tend to come with the wear and tear of time. Firmer muscles means improved shape, and there is usually a reduction of fat in the hips, thighs, waist, chin and neck.

The improved blood supply to the internal organs improves their functioning, further boosted by the action on the endocrine system. The whole central nervous system is stimulated along with the autonomic nervous system.

The spine becomes more flexible and strong, backache (we hope!) becomes a stranger as the vertebrae are realigned (and when you think that nearly everyone suffers backache at some time, this is no small thing).

Individual âsanas

Let's take a look at the benefits of the individual âsanas.

Samasthiti: The body is brought to attention and any imbalances in posture can be spotted and corrected—for example, sway-back can be corrected by consciously tilting the pelvis. Having the feet and palms of the hands together creates circuits which allow bio-energy to flow freely, inducing calmness and activating *anâhata chakra*, the heart centre.

Hasta uttânâsana: Backward extension of the spine stimulates the spinal nerves and spongy discs, as well as the sympathetic and parasympathetic nervous systems, situated along the spine. Lung capacity is increased by the opening of the ribcage and arching back helps to drain the nasal passages. The abdominal muscles are stretched and toned, improving digestion, and excess fat is reduced, partly by the stretch and because the thyroid gland is stimulated as the neck lengthens backward. The muscles and ligaments of the arms are toned, and any roundness of the shoulders is lessened.

Pâdahastâsana: All the muscles of the back and of the backs of the legs are stretched and toned, as well as the wrist muscles. The abdominal organs are massaged, improving digestion and elimination and toning the reproductive organs. There is an increase in the flow of freshly-oxygenated blood to the brain, the facial tissues and hair follicles. The pituitary and pineal glands in the brain and thyroid and parathyroid glands in the neck also receive fresh blood.

Aśwa sanchalanâsana: The lower back and the

muscles of the fronts of the legs are toned. The pelvic region and its organs are stimulated. The glands in the neck are again worked, this time by stretching backward. The stretch to the abdominal area tones the pancreas and liver, while the stretching of the perineal muscles eases any menstrual tension and is helpful in pregnancy too.

Pârśvottânâsana: The muscles and joints of the hips and shoulders are toned and become more supple, and the whole spine is stretched. The abdominal massage afforded by bringing the body to the thighs tones the digestive system as all the abdominal organs are contracted, toned and stimulated.

Trikonâsana: The ankle and leg muscles and the hips are toned and strengthened, and backache is relieved. The neck muscles are also toned, and the chest opened as the intercostal muscles are developed.

Parivrrta trikonâsana: Here you have all the benefits of the previous pose plus an increased blood supply to the lower back. The whole back is given a spiral stretch that releases tension and eases backache and helps to realign the spine. This includes the neck region, so it is particularly useful in combating stress-related neck problems.

Santolanâsana: The arms, wrists and shoulders are toned and strengthened; the back is stretched gently.

Bhujangâsana: The opening of the chest renders the intercostal muscles supple, which in turn facilitates better breathing, This posture stretches the anterior face of the spine and has even been known to replace slipped discs. It improves the circulation in the back, tones the nerves, the reproductive organs, liver, kidneys and adrenal glands. The arms and wrists are strengthened and toned, and by bringing together the shoulder blades, tension stored under them is dispersed.

Adho mukha śvânâsana: Not only the hamstring muscles and back knee-tendons, but also the calf muscles and Achilles tendons receive a good stretch. Both legs and arms, especially the wrists, are strengthened, and the whole back stretched, especially the sacral spine and the sciatic nerve. The neck muscles are released. Because of the full stretch of the back, the whole spine is extended agreeably, opening up the spaces between the vertebrae, releasing spinal nerves and activating all the energy centres along the spine. A good flow of blood to the brain, facial tissues and hair follicles promotes rejuvenation—something yoga is renowned for!

Konâsana: Lifting the head and keeping the neck long strengthens the neck muscles and tones the thyroid gland; drawing the shoulder blades down opens the chest and improves the breathing.

Along with these physical benefits, there are more subtle benefits. Your concentration is improved and this brings a calmer mind and a feeling of peace, of well-being. Awareness is improved too and subtle energy channels (*nâdîs*) unblock so that energy can flow freely in your body.

Whatever the present condition of your body, it has taken years to achieve; any problem you have has had plenty of time to develop and settle into place, so you can't reasonably expect a change overnight. You won't get a revolution with yoga because yoga works to evolve. Sri Aurobindo said, 'yoga is condensed evolution'.

Stiffness is due to tension—or sometimes sheer bulk—in the muscles, or to tightness of tendons or ligaments, or to toxic deposits in the joints. Tension is released through conscious relaxation, and toxic deposits will be cleared gradually with regular practice and attention to what you eat. As I said, this is the only body you have and you're going to be in it right to the end, so never fight with your body; listen to it, learn to harmonize with it.

If you're in doubt about anything, find a qualified yoga teacher and ask advice before joining the class. And if you don't like it, try another—yoga teachers are not factory produced, they are not identical! And there are many different styles of yoga (one size does not fit all!), so there's sure to be one that suits your needs. If you have a specific problem there are teachers trained to give specialist help.

In practising, remember the following golden rules:

Never force your body into a posture, simply invite it to accompany you there.

Never go so far that stretch turns to pain. The more you relax into a stretch, the better the stretch.

Remain positive in your approach—even if you couldn't do this posture yesterday, you may be able to do it tomorrow, or next week, or next year. There's no hurry….

CHAPTER FOUR:
THE HISTORY OF SÛRYA NAMASKÂR

OUR EARLY ancestors were well tuned to their environment—they had to be in order to survive. They were acutely aware of the powers of the forces of nature and realized that the earth provides us with sustenance, and the energy that permits all life on our planet emanates from the sun. The turning of the seasons, the effects of the weather, even the moods of the individual—all are linked to the amount of heat and light from the sun. And, as humankind is wont to do, our ancestors feared and admired this power, and deified it. In all parts of our planet, of all the forms of nature that have been worshipped, the sun has been the most revered. Even today, in what we consider to be 'enlightened times', the sun is respected as the source of light, life, and energy.

Apart from the millions of people who go to enormous expense and effort to worship the sun on beaches, on boats, beside pools, etc., there are also the scientists and inventors who seek to harness the sun's rays to produce heat, light and motive power for our immediate use, as well as all those who are investigating its future applications.

But to return to our ancestors: it's easy to find evidence of sun worship in the artefacts and architecture of ancient civilizations, and in stories that have been handed down throughout history. In India, the early yogis revered the sun and daily performed rites in reverence to it. These rites are known to have involved throwing water at the sun's rays, the use of incense, flowers, fire, camphor, the recitation of prayers and of *mantras*, deep breathing, gesticulations and prostrations.

Yogis of old may not have had doctorates in anatomy and physiology, but they knew a lot about the body. For example, they knew of the existence of the endocrine and exocrine glands and their importance in general health, and they also knew that some of these glands are photoactive. They knew that sunshine can be harmful but that early morning and late evening sunshine is beneficial, so *sûrya namaskâr* involved exposure to the early morning rays.

Originally, *pranâm mudrâ* began at the chest and moved up to the throat, the forehead, the crown of the head, then up to the sky (thus incorporating the upper *chakra*s, the centres of energy in the body and the aura). There was the symbolism of touching the sky and the earth, acknowledging Man's dependence on the sun as source of all life energy, and the Earth which manifests that energy. There was a full prostration along the ground, face down, with the arms extended above the head as an act of submission to the highest power of the universe—these days if present at all this is abridged to a quick knees-chest-chin-on-the-ground. There were also deep squats, and in the semi-kneeling position the arms were thrown back in a 'sunburst breath' which is omitted in the majority of modern versions.

Sûrya namaskâr was always performed slowly and with deep concentration and devotion, and *mantra*s were recited either verbally or mentally. The sequence evolved gradually into an efficient training of the mind and body but not as part of the yoga tradition. It remained a part of the worship rites and also became a discipline of the body. As such it was adopted for use by the warrior caste, the *Kṣatriyas*, to improve strength, suppleness and concentration. In the epic story, the *Ramâyana*, the sage Viśvâmitra taught it to Râma to strengthen him in battle against Râvana, a foe of far greater strength and superior martial ability and experience—with excellent results.

It remained unknown in the West until Balasaheb Pant Pratinidhi, the Rajah of Aundh, published his book *Sûrya Namaskâr: the Ten-point Way to Health* in 1928. Later Swami Sivananda Saraśwati popularised another version known as the Rishikesh *sûrya namaskâr*. This has featured in many books on yoga. Many yoga teachers in the West teach it, often (unfortunately) merely as a warm-up sequence and even at night.

Humankind has evolved beyond mere worship of the forces of Nature and can perceive the divinity beyond the sun. Nevertheless the sun remains the largest and most obvious manifestation of the creative force and can still serve as a focus for meditation or appreciation of the Creator and of creation.

Unlike *sûrya namaskâr*, *chandra namaskâr* is a sequence that has evolved inside the yoga tradition—and very recently. I have come across several different sequences so far, but have chosen the one given in the next chapter for its completeness and the way it differs so much from *sûrya namaskâr*.

CHAPTER FIVE: SALUTATION TO THE MOON

BY EVENING, larks are beginning to feel less energetic and are more or less winding down for the day, waiting for the moment when they can 'get horizontal'. Early evening is a good time for them to do *chandra namaskâr*, the Salute to the Moon, which will revive them enough to get them through the evening. Owls too can practise and enjoy this sequence and will probably find it easy to do, being so much more supple in the evening.

In western cultures, the moon was always seen as feminine. As the sister of the sun god, she was known by many names—Luna, Selene, Artemis, Diana, or Phoebe. Yet in many ancient cultures such as India, Egypt, Mesopotamia and South America, the moon is considered to be a masculine deity. In India the male deity of the moon is Chandra (which means 'shining, bright').

The moon has a powerful effect on the Earth's tides, and as we are about seventy per cent water ourselves, you can imagine that the moon has an effect on our energies and on our emotions, over a monthly cycle. (The Latin word *mensis*, a month, gives us 'menses' and 'menstruation'.) Because the moon moves around the Earth in an ellipse, it appears to change in shape and size, and its effects vary in strength because of this elliptical trajectory. Moreover the effects can vary on individuals. Once, people even believed that the human brain shrank in size with the waning moon and re-grew with the waxing moon!

A subtle change in energies can be observed with the time of month you practise this sequence. Around the time of the new moon, you may notice that the energy produced induces calm, whereas around the time of the full moon the energy is much more tonic, especially if the full moon coincides with the perigee, when it is closest to the Earth.

As a fair amount of this sequence is on one knee, it's advisable to have a soft mat. If your mat is not thick enough, place a folded towel under your knees for extra protection. If your knees are particularly fragile, place the extra padding under the shins, leaving the knees free.

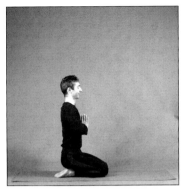

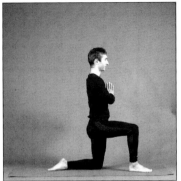

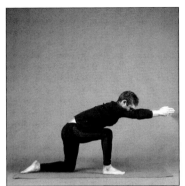

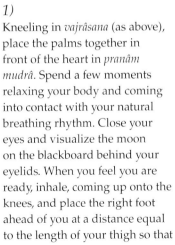

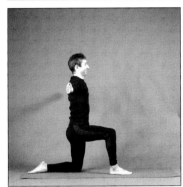

1)

Kneeling in *vajrâsana* (as above), place the palms together in front of the heart in *pranâm mudrâ*. Spend a few moments relaxing your body and coming into contact with your natural breathing rhythm. Close your eyes and visualize the moon on the blackboard behind your eyelids. When you feel you are ready, inhale, coming up onto the knees, and place the right foot ahead of you at a distance equal to the length of your thigh so that there's a right angle at the knee.

2)

Then, exhaling (*mûla bandha*), lean forward, stretching forward with both arms (palms together) until the whole upper body is parallel to the floor. The right ischium (sitting bone) is aiming towards the right heel. If knee injury makes this unwise, keep the shin vertical.

3)

Inhale, returning to upright, and stretch the arms out sideways at shoulder height, keeping the shoulders relaxed and down, and the spine long. (The right shin

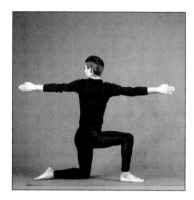 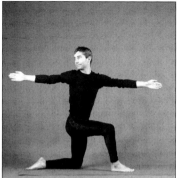 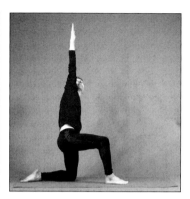

and the left thigh are vertical.)

4)

Exhale (*mûla bandha*) as you turn the whole upper body to the left, turning the head to look at the left thumb.

5)

Inhale as you return to the front, keeping the spine extended, especially the neck.

6)

Exhale (*mûla bandha*) as you twist

the upper body to the right, turning the head gently to look at the right thumb. Try to keep the arms at shoulder level but without letting the shoulders lift towards the ears—bring the shoulder blades together and down to facilitate this.

7)

Inhale as you return to the front.

8)

Exhaling, lean sideways and place the left hand on the floor,

either flat or on the tips of the fingers (*mûla bandha*). Stretch the right hand up towards the sky to open the chest, keeping the neck long and turning the head gently to look up at the thumb. Make sure the head remains aligned with the spine and does not drop towards the shoulder.

9)

Inhale as you return to vertical, the arms still outstretched and the face forward.

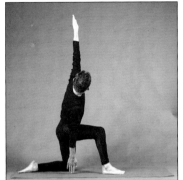

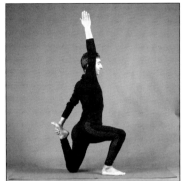

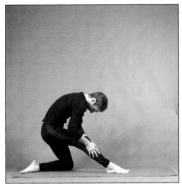

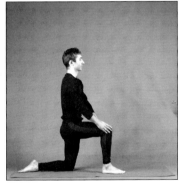

floor (*mûla bandha*). Stretch the left hand up towards the sky to open the chest, turning the head gently to look up at the thumb.

11)

This time, as you inhale, place both hands on the right knee. Here comes the tricky bit….

12)

…as you exhale (*mûla bandha*), move the hips forward as if to sit on the right heel and, keeping the upper body vertical, stretch the right hand forward horizontally,

then lift the left foot off the ground and catch it with the left hand.

13)

Inhale as you lift the right hand to vertical and (if possible) look up at the thumb. I say if possible because there's quite a large element of balance in this movement. Try to keep both the breath and the movements fluid to help maintain your balance.

14)

Exhale (*mûla bandha*), bring both hands onto the right shin and

10)

Exhale as you lean to the right and place the right hand on the

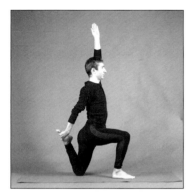
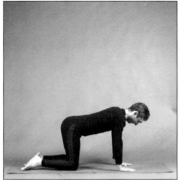
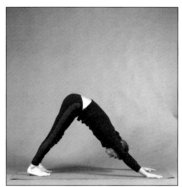

draw the hips back as if about to sit on the left heel. This stretches out the spine and releases any tension in the lower back and in the right leg. Relax.

15)

Inhale as you reach up with the left hand this time and lift the left foot. Catch the left foot with the right hand. Although this resembles (13) it will feel very different!

16)

Retain your breath (*antar*

kumbhaka) and come down to all fours into *marjariâsana,* the cat pose; relax the back and keep the head in line with the spine. Feel a stretch from the coccyx right along the spine to the crown of the head.

17)

Exhale (*mûla bandha*) and straighten both legs, lifting the hips high and lowering the heels, coming into *adho mukha śvânâsana,* the down-facing dog pose, and lengthen the whole

spine as you lift the shoulders away from the wrists and the hips away from the shoulders. Look at the knees to ensure the neck remains relaxed. Ideally the heels are almost in contact with the floor in order to leave some room for stretch.

18) (photograph overleaf)

Breathe at your own speed for these next few movements: still in down-facing dog, lift the right leg as high as you can, keeping the leg straight. Feel the stretch from

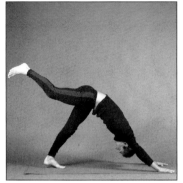

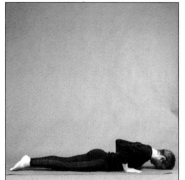

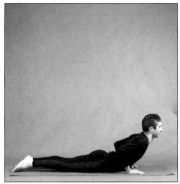

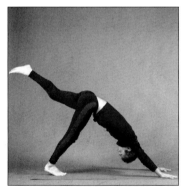

the fingertips to the tips of the toes in a long, diagonal line.

19)
Replace the foot beside the left one; verify all the elements of the down-facing dog pose, then….

20)
…. lift the left leg as high as you comfortably can. Again feel the diagonal line stretch.

21)
Return to the down-facing dog, check all the elements and ensure the neck (and face!) are still relaxed.

22)
Inhale as you swoop down and forwards by bending the elbows, to come into *bhujangâsana*, the cobra. Keep the nape of the neck long, the shoulders down, the elbows close to the ribs, and the face vertical—a cobra stares straight ahead in order to hypnotise its prey. To protect the lumbar spine it's a good idea to press the pubic bone gently against the mat. This tilts the pelvis and lengthens the lower back.

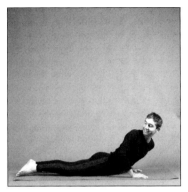

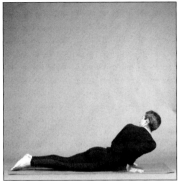

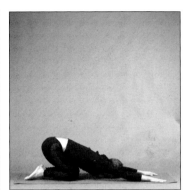

23)

Exhale (*mûla bandha*) as you turn the head to the right as if to look at the left heel (yes, I did say left heel, but I also said 'as if'!).

24)

Inhale, bringing the face forward and checking the relaxation in the shoulders, neck and face.

25)

Exhale (*mûla bandha*), turning the head to the left as if to see the right heel—which you may do if your shoulders are sufficiently relaxed.

26)

Inhale, turning the face forward.

27)

Exhale (*mûla bandha*), as you come onto all fours and (you'll like this bit!) in one fluid and graceful movement, sit back down on the heels in *sâdhakâsana*. Relax the whole back and the shoulders. Feel the gentle pressure of the mat on the forehead at *âjnâ chakra*. You may feel like taking an extra breath in this posture as it's so relaxing.

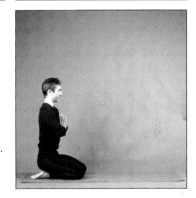

28)

Inhale as you return to *vajrâsana* with the hands in *pranâm mudrâ*.

Now you're ready to repeat the whole procedure leading with the left leg to complete the sequence. Afterwards, just as with the *sûrya namaskâr* in the morning, take a few minutes to rest in *śavâsana* or to meditate, and consciously follow your breathing. And notice how you feel invigorated and refreshed.

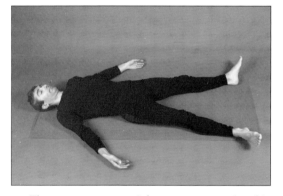

There are twenty-eight movements in this sequence, just as there are twenty-eight days in the lunar cycle. But you don't have to do the sequence twenty-eight times to get any benefits from it (whew!). This sequence presents you with a complete practice as it comprises concentration on the breath, forward and backward bends, lateral stretches, twists, an inversion and even an element of balance. So you get the benefits of all the various elements as in *sûrya namaskâr* but with different movements.

Now go back to Chapter Three, 'After the *Namaskâr*', to read about rest and relaxation following the sequence. What is says applies equally after the *chandra namaskâr*.

Benefits of the Postures

You want the individual posture benefits explained? Okay, here goes:

1) *Vajrâsana* tones the abdominal organs and improves digestion (you can practise this posture after a meal). It also tones the pelvic muscles and renders the knees and ankles supple. It strengthens the spine and helps to realign it in cases of lordosis and scoliosis. Lastly, it relieves varicose veins, improving the circulation to the legs and feet.

2) The spine is stretched and neural pathways liberated between the discs; the neck muscles are toned and strengthened; the lungs are stretched and toned. The ascending colon is stimulated in the first part of the sequence, the descending colon during the second part when you lead with the left

leg, thus improving digestion and elimination.

3) Again, the ribcage is opened and the intercostal muscles toned, improving respiration generally.

4) This gentle twist tones the back muscles and limbers the spinal column.

6) As for (4) but accentuated.

8) The spine is limbered and the chest opened; the kidneys are toned and also the stomach; the right lung is stretched and the left one massaged, stimulating and toning the respiratory system.

10) This time the liver is toned, the left lung stretched and the right lung massaged.

12) The lumbar spine is toned and the kidneys massaged; the left thigh is stretched.

13) As (12) though accentuated by the upward stretch of the arm; the right shoulder is toned.

14) The spine is gently stretched and eased, the right leg also.

15) As (13) with the left shoulder toned.

16) This posture relaxes the back and releases any tension in the abdominal area.

17), 19) and 21) All the benefits of this posture are already explained in the section on *sûrya namaskâr*.

18) and (20) As (17) except that raising a leg increases the stretch along one side of the torso and the leg itself, and facilitates venous return.

22), 24) and 25) *bhujangâsana* opens the chest to facilitate better breathing, it stretches the anterior face of the spine and has even been known to replace slipped discs. It improves the circulation in the back, tones the nerves, the reproductive organs, liver, kidneys and adrenal glands.

23) and 25) Add a slight upper body twist to the cobra and you have toning of the upper back and accentuated effects on the digestive system. The eye muscles and the optic nerve are also toned here.

27) The delightful stretch and release of the whole back in *sâdhakâsana* releases pressure on the discs. The toning of the shoulders and upper back results in relaxation of this part of the body where we tend to stock tension. It tones the reproductive and digestive organs.

CHAPTER SIX: ON MANTRA, THE POWER OF SOUND

SOUND IS vibration; it can create forms and affect them. Every movement creates a sound, sometimes beyond our normal hearing range, and sounds may be beneficial, neutral or detrimental. The most obvious example is music: we all have favourite pieces of music which make us feel happy, nostalgic or whatever, and who hasn't experienced some discomfort when subjected to a noisy neighbour's choice or to the muzak in public places? In our ancestors' days the bard was rated on his ability to transform the emotions of his listeners, and the sixteenth-century Indian musician Tansen became a legend for stopping a drought by singing up a rainstorm. The walls of Jericho were destroyed by trumpet blasts (I wonder what they did to everyone's eardrums?), and using a sonar scanner you can see an unborn baby in the womb. So you can see that sound has power, and this power has been studied by yogis for centuries, the results of which are: *mantra*.

Mantras come in many forms. They are classified as being male or female, sun or moon, and so on, while at the same time they are either *kanthika* (throated—that is, audible) or *ajapa* (not uttered). *Kanthika mantra*s may be spoken aloud, 'hummed' or whispered. An *ajapa mantra* can be either silent and visualized in its Sanskrit form, or meditated upon by mental repetition. A *mantra* has great power if transmitted orally by a guru, but is considered by some (especially by those who sell them) to have no practical value if learned from a book.

Mantras are often the concentrated essence of a great deal of wisdom and stories are told of people overhearing a *mantra* being given as initiation to a pupil by a guru, and the eavesdropper (in the stories this is usually an illiterate peasant) attaining enlightenment as if he'd spent years studying the secret doctrine. Now is that power, or what?

Sanskrit is considered to be the most perfect of languages. It has fifty letters in its alphabet and, unlike most languages, it is spoken as it is written (which simplifies things a lot). Sanskrit pronunciation is standardized and correct pronunciation is considered vital in *mantra japa*. You hear awful stories of dire things befalling those who mispronounce their *mantra*s! While there is more than a possibility that these are in the same vein as the apocryphal stories and urban myths common in the West, it's still a good idea to try and get it right, just in case! Ideally, you'll be able to find a yoga teacher who has studied Sanskrit and can ensure you've got it right. Meanwhile, perhaps the following will help.

The Vowels

a—short, as in *organ*
i—short, as in *pin*
u—short, as in *bush*
e—long, as in *they*
o—as in *go*

â—long, as in *far*
î—long, like *ee* in *seek*
û—long, as in *rule*
ai—as in *aisle*
au—ow, as in *how*

Special Consonants

m—resonates in the nose like the *n* in the French word *bon*.

h—the final *h* is always aspirated and more like 'ha', so *namah* is pronounced 'namaha'.

Where you find *bh* and *kh*, you pronounce them b-h and k-h (as in *cub-hat*; *book-house*).

Pronounce 'r' by flicking the tongue tip against the front of the palate.

There are three kinds of s in Sanskrit:
s—as in *sun*
ś—as in *shine*, and
ṣ—which is somewhere between the two.

Using mantras

There are several options for using *mantra*s with *sûrya namaskâr*. Which method you choose will depend on how long you wish to spend chanting, on how alert you feel—chanting gives you energy and a respite between rounds for the body to settle—and on how many rounds you plan to do. Some people prefer to repeat the *mantra* mentally; in this case the physical benefits of the *mantra*s are rendered much more subtle and less physical. If you choose to chant aloud, you chant the *mantra* clearly and audibly, and retain the sound of it in your mind's ear.

• You can chant *OM* with a solar *mantra* at the start of each round, progressing through all the twelve solar *mantra*s—for which, see below.

• You can chant a *bîja mantra* (also set out below) at the start of each round, or while holding each posture, or four times at the end of each round.

• You can chant the six *bîja mantra*s at the start of each round.

• You can chant all twelve *mantra*s at the start of *sûrya namaskâr*.

The Solar Mantras
for use with sûrya namaskâr

aum hrâm mitrâya namah
(om hraam mitraaya namaha)
Salutations to the Friend of all.

aum hrîm ravaye namah
(om hreem ravayey namaha)
Salutations to the Shining One.

aum hrûm sûryâya namah
(om hroom sooryaaya namaha)
Salutations to the One who induces activity.

aum hraim bhânave namah
(om hraim b-haanavey namaha)
Salutations to the Diffuser of Light.

aum hraum khagâya namah
(om hrowm k-hagaaya namaha)
Salutations to the One who moves in the sky.

aum hrâh pûśne namah
(om hraaha pooshney namaha)
Salutations to the Nourisher of Life.

aum hrâm hiranyagharbâya namah
(om hraam hiranya garb-haaya namaha)
Salutations to that which contains everything.

aum hrîm marîchâye namah
(om hreem mareechaayey namaha)
Salutations to the One possessing rays.

aum hrûm âdityâya namah
(om hroom aadityaaya namaha)
Salutations to the One who inspires love.

aum hraim savitre namah
(om hraim savitrey namaha)
Salutations to the Begetter of Life.

aum hraum arkâya namah
(om hrowm arkaaya namaha)
Salutations to the One fit to be praised.

aum hrah bhâskarâya namah
(om hraha b-haaskaraaya namaha)
Salutations to the One who leads to Enlightenment.

The Bîja Mantras

The vibrations of the *bîja* ('seed') *mantra*s have a powerful effect on the body. The *bîja mantra*s used for *sûrya namaskâr* are all single syllables starting with 'h'—this is aspirated and comes from the heart. The 'r' vibrates the brain. Most of them end with 'm' which clears the nasal passages, facilitating respiration, in turn improving the quality of the blood.

'Hrâm' works on the upper three pairs of ribs and stimulates the apical lobes of the lungs, helping to fight against respiratory problems such as asthma and bronchitis.

'Hrîm' vibrates the throat, palate, nose, and the right and left auricles of the heart, working to clear the respiratory and digestive passages of phlegm.

'Hrûm' works on the abdominal organs, particularly the liver, spleen, uterus, stomach and intestines.

'Hraim' promotes urination by working on the kidneys.

'Hraum' stimulates the rectum and the anus; if you haven't defecated already, then don't be surprised if you get a bowel movement about half an hour after your practice.

'Hrah', the only one to lack an 'm', works on the throat and the whole chest area.

Om

Just as light passing through a prism will emerge as a rainbow, so the sound of *OM* passing through the prism of the space-time continuum is said to emerge as all other sounds. *OM* is analyzed as A-U-M. 'A' begins at the solar plexus; it is the first letter of the alphabet, it is the state of waking consciousness, it is the beginning. It evolves upward to the back of the throat where it becomes 'U', the state of dreaming consciousness. It rises, flows along the tongue and arrives at the teeth, becoming a labial sound—'M', the third state, that of sleeping consciousness. This humming rolls up through the nose, becomes a cerebral sound and leaves the body via the top of the skull, now beyond all letters and becomes supreme consciousness, devoid of duality. *OM* precedes all other *mantra*s. On the mundane level, it regulates and develops the action of the heart.

The Lunar Mantras
for use with chandra namaskâr

The lunar *mantra*s address the female aspect of God. They accompany the practice to render it more profound and spiritual, and are usually chanted at the beginning of each round. Practice of any kind of *sâdhanâ* is considered to be enhanced when started at the beginning of a lunar month, when the celestial orb begins to wax. One *mantra* is chanted on the first evening, the second *mantra* on the second, and so on until full moon, then one begins again with the first *mantra*. It's interesting to observe how one's energy can change with the waxing and waning of the moon, and I must say this is much more easily observed under clear skies when you can actually see the moon while you practise.

Om kameśwarai namaha
Salutations to the goddess of desire.

Om bhagamalinyai namaha
Salutations to the one wearing the garland of prosperity.

Om nityaklinnayai namaha
Salutations to the one who is infinitely compassionate.

Om bherundi namaha
Salutations to the terrible one.

Om vahnivasinyai namaha
Salutations to the controller of fire.

Om vajeśwarai namaha
Salutations to the mighty one.

Om śivaduti namaha
Salutations to the messenger of Shiva.

Om tvaritai namaha
Salutations to the speedy one.

Om kalasundari namaha
Salutations to the sweet and beautiful one.

Om nityai namaha
Salutations to the everlasting one.

Om nîlapatakayai namaha
Salutations to the carrier of the blue flag.

Om vijayai namaha
Salutations to the victorious one.

Om sarvamangalyai namaha
Salutations to the auspicious one.

Om jvalamalinyai namaha
Salutations to the one wearing the garland of fire.

CHAPTER SEVEN: THE BREATH OF LIFE

The nose is a wonderfully complex instrument, far better suited to dealing with the breath than is the mouth. If you have a cold or catarrh, it's well worth spending a little time cleansing the nasal passages before you begin your practice. There are several ways to do this, apart from the time-honoured method of blowing your nose (which, as you probably know, you should do one nostril at a time in order not to put undue pressure on the Eustachian tubes to the ears).

Ardha padadirâsana:

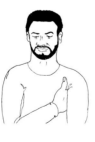

If a nostril is blocked, tuck the (same side) hand under the armpit of the opposite, i.e. unblocked side, and breathe smoothly and deeply for a few minutes; the blocked nostril will clear quite quickly. If both nostrils are blocked, tuck both hands under the opposite armpits.

Vama Krama

Form the fingers of the right hand into *Vishnu mudrâ* by curling the forefinger and middle fingers down to the palm and secure them with the root of the thumb. Close the right nostril just below the bony part with the thumb and inhale softly through the left nostril. Close the left nostril with the third finger (supported by the little finger) and exhale softly through the right nostril; inhale through the same nostril before closing it with the thumb, then open the left nostril and exhale. This is one round. Start off slowly and speed up with successive rounds, then slow down again—it will sound like a steam train accelerating and slowing down, and is affectionately known to my students as the 'choo-choo breath'. But who cares what it's called? It works! Note that it is the momentum that alters, not the force!

Sorry, left-handers, traditionally it has to be the right hand because in India the left hand is used for below-the-belt cleansing only!

Jala neti

Dissolve a pinch of salt in a bowl of lukewarm water (at a ratio of 1:100 which works out at a teaspoonful for half a litre), and pour some of it into your cupped hand. Lukewarm is good; the warmer the water, the faster it loosens the mucus, and the cooler the water, the more it toughens. Sniff the water up one nostril, keeping the other closed, and let the water run down the back of the nose into the mouth, then spit it out into a second bowl or the sink. Repeat several times then repeat the process with the other nostril. In persistent cases of catarrh or with sinusitis you can sniff up the water, tip the head forward holding both nostrils closed, and roll the head from side to side to rinse out all the nooks and crannies. If you have a neti pot, simply pour the water through one nostril and let it flow out through the other, then repeat the procedure via the other nostril. For stubborn mucus, sniffing up the water from the hand is more effective.

Always sit for a few moments after emptying both nostrils to let the sinuses drain before doing *vâma krama* (see above) to dry them out thoroughly.

Remember that dairy products tend to increase the mucus production in the body, so if you're plagued with catarrh or sinusitis, you could try cutting back on milk and cheese for a while.

CHAPTER EIGHT: THE PRECEPTS OF YOGA

Traditionally the precepts of Yoga constitute the 'first steps' on the Yogic path. While most westerners ignore them, they remain an important step worthy of your consideration. These rules refer here to your practice but can, perhaps even should, be broadened to include your whole lifestyle, and to affect your attitude to life and Creation.

YAMA: the rules of conduct

1) ahimsâ: non-violence

Remain mindful of your body while doing your *sûrya* or *chandra namaskâr* and ensure you don't ignore this first precept by harming your body—or your emotions. Don't allow yourself to get carried away! You can be a pacifist vegetarian and still abuse *ahimsâ* by being cruel to yourself, so make sure this starts from the inside. Don't overdo it, don't criticize yourself. Keep away from negativity.

2) satya: truthfulness

Are you being honest with yourself in your practice? Do you ever indulge in maybe a hint of self-deception occasionally?

3) asteya: non-stealing

So you're not the neighbourhood burglar, but have you ever taken the credit for someone else's idea? Have you ever taken over somebody's project? Stealing can be a very subtle activity—be your own Thought Police.

4) brahmacharya: continence

Some take this to mean complete sexual abstinence, which is fine if you're a natural monk or nun; otherwise it means not to waste energy through sensuality. The endless (and unfulfillable) search for Pleasure is only the search for one's inner Self in disguise.

5) aparigraha: coveting

This is linked with no. (2) in the *niyamas* below, as when you are content with your lot in life, you tend not to covet another's lot (or part thereof). But also it's useless to covet in other ways. For example, if today your *sûrya namaskâr* is more difficult because your body seems stiffer than yesterday, it's a complete waste of energy to wish it to be like it was yesterday.

NIYAMA: the rules of inner control

1) *śaucha:* purity of mind and body.
You've probably already noticed that what you eat, drink, hear, watch, read, etc., affect you deeply. Sooner or later you'll feel like cleaning up your act to clean up your Self. Remember that the body is a vehicle; would you treat your car like this? How well do you treat your car—do you fill it with cheapo fuel and oil? Do you have the car serviced regularly and do you keep the tyres at the right pressure? How well do you treat your body? Apply the same criteria…. You can buy a new car but you can't buy a new body! Moreover, the purer and more biogenic your diet, the less stiffness you'll experience in your joints.

2) *santoṣa:* contentment
Be happy with what you have; the alternative is constant hankering after things difficult to achieve. What waste of energy! What an invitation to suffering!

3) *tapas:* austerity
I could tell you stories of yogis who took this very literally and to extremes. But there's no need for extremes in life, is there? A certain amount of self-discipline is all you need to get you up and out and doing your *sûrya namaskâr* daily—the benefits follow automatically. Consider *tapas* as the search for simplicity in your life, and try not to overindulge in any way.

4) *svâdhyâya:* self-study
No, not involving a mirror! Watch how the real You begins to shine through with your regular practice. Keep your attention on what is needed and don't allow it to wander; during your practice be wholly aware, let your consciousness fill your body like your hand fills a glove.

5) *îśvara pranidhâna:* devotion to God
This is the one that trips up all the atheists, agnostics and Buddhists, so if this includes you—you're not alone. But yoga is not a religion, doing *sûrya* or *chandra namaskâr* is not sun-worship, and whatever your system of belief, *sûrya* and *chandra namaskâr* will tend to strengthen it as your practice brings your mind/body/spirit into balance and harmony. We are all part of Creation; real awareness of this fact brings us into harmony with the rest of Creation.

GLOSSARY

âjnâ chakra: the 'Third Eye', or Command Centre, is located at the cavernous plexus in the forehead. Its symbol is a white triangle and it is connected with intuition and thought. Its *bîja mantra* is *aum*.

anâhata chakra: the Heart Centre, located at the cardiac plexus. This is the Air Centre and governs touch. Its symbol is a smoky blue six-pointed star. Its *bîja mantra* is *yam*.

âsana: literally means 'seat', but here means posture.

bandha: literally means a confinement; a technique of contraction or compression to pressurise *prâna* and control it.

bîja: a seed

brahma muhurta: the 'Brahmin hour'. Actually a two-hour period preceding and including sunrise when the earth is quiet and its energies neutral, so a good time for meditation.

chakra: literally means a wheel. These are energy vortices in the body located at the intersections of energy channels (*nâdîs*). Of the thousands found in the subtle body, the most important (those listed here) correspond loosely to major nerve plexi in the physical body.

chandra: the moon

dhâranâ : concentration or complete awareness.

guna: a quality of nature. There are three : *tamas*, *rajas* and *sattva* (which see).

hatha yoga: the branch of yoga concerned mainly with physical disciplines and respiration to prepare the body and mind for *raja yoga* and meditation. *Ha* (sun) and *tha* (moon) energies are balanced and merged resulting in yoga (unison).

îda nâdî : the subtle channel for lunar, cool, passive energy, and linked to the parasympathetic nervous system. It is dominant when the breath flows more strongly through the left nostril.

jâla neti: water irrigation of the nasal passages. See the chapter, 'The Breath of Life'.

kośa: a sheath. There are five sheaths that make up the human being: *annamayakośa*, the physical layer, *prânâmayakośa*, the energy layer, *manomayakośa*, the mind layer, *vijnânamayakośa*, the intuitive layer, and *anandamayakośa*, the layer of bliss.

kumbhaka: the interval of time between inhalation and exhalation, known as *antar kumbhaka*; or between exhalation and inhalation, known as *bahya kumbhaka*.

manas: the higher or thinking part of the mind, the ruler of the senses.

manipûra chakra : the energy vortex situated at the solar plexus, this is the Fire Centre and governs sight. Its symbol is a red triangle and its *bîja mantra* is *ram*.

mantra : a word, syllable or phrase containing the concentrated essence of much hidden wisdom.

mâyâ: illusion, specifically that which lets us think the Universe is real and separate from the Supreme Spirit.

mudrâ: a seal or gesture.

mûla bandha: the 'root lock', one of the three major contractions. The tightening of the muscles of the pelvic floor, or more correctly the anterior sphincter, to control *prâna* in the lower body. This is effected after full exhalation, and is always released before inhalation.

mûlâdhâra chakra: the Root Chakra, situated at the base of the spine between the anal orifice and the genital organs in the perineum. It is the earth centre and is related to smell. Its symbol is a yellow square, its *bîja mantra* is *lam*.

nâdî: there are 72,000 *nâdîs* or energy channels in the body. The three principal are *idâ, pingalâ,* and *suṣumnâ*; they are situated along the spine and terminate respectively at the left nostril, the right nostril, and the *sutura frontalis* at the top of the head. They intersect at major energy centres (the *chakra*s).

namaskâr: greeting, salutation.

prâna: breath, energy, especially bio-energy or life-force.

pingalâ nadî: the subtle channel for solar, dynamic, extravert energy linked to the sympathetic nervous system. It is dominant when the breath flows more freely through the right nostril.

puraka: inhalation.

rajas: activity, passion. One of the three constituents of nature.

rechaka: exhalation.

sâdhakâsana: the adept's pose. This posture relaxes the whole spine and the head.

sâdhanâ: practice, spiritual discipline.

sahasrâra chakra: the 'Thousand-Petalled Lotus'. This energy vortex is situated just above the top of the head. Its element is spirit, its symbol, the thousand-petalled lotus.

samasthiti âsana: *sama* means equal, balanced; *sthiti* means firm.

sattva: purity, the illuminating quality of nature.

śavâsana: the Corpse Posture. This *âsana* produces deep relaxation and is always performed after a session of yoga to relax both the body and the mind.

sûrya: the Sun.

suṣumnâ nâdî: the central and most important of the subtle energy channels, linking all the *chakra*s and directing energy to higher levels for the attainment of Oneness.

svâdhiṣthâna chakra: this energy vortex is situated at the pelvic plexus and relates to the element water. It governs taste and its symbol is a white crescent. The *bîja mantra* is *vam*.

uddiyâna bandha: the 'flying up' lock. The contraction and lifting of the abdominal muscles to control *prâna* in the middle body.

vajrâsana: *vajra* means thunderbolt or diamond.

viśuddha chakra: the energy vortex situated at the laryngeal plexus in the throat. Its element is ether and it governs the sense of hearing. Its symbol is a white circle and the *bîja mantra* is *ham*.

Yogi: one who practises yoga (male).

Yogini: one who practises yoga (female).

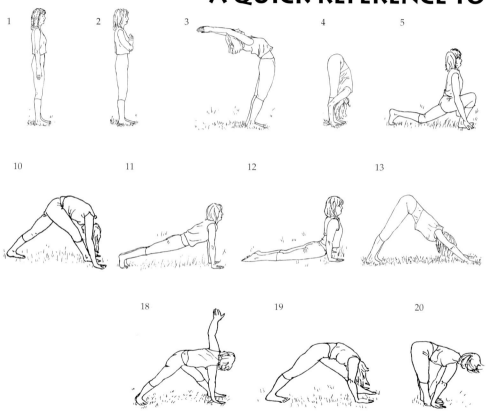

1 2 3 4 5

10 11 12 13

18 19 20

SÛRYA NAMASKÂR

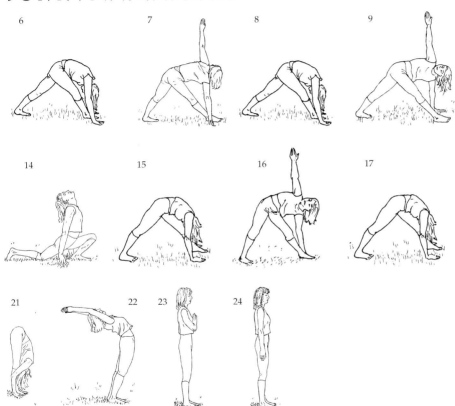

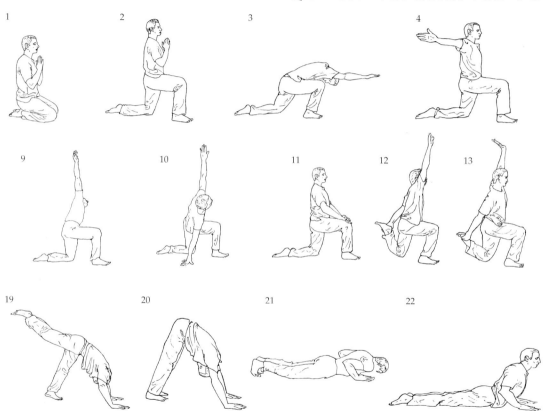

CHANDRA NAMASKÂR

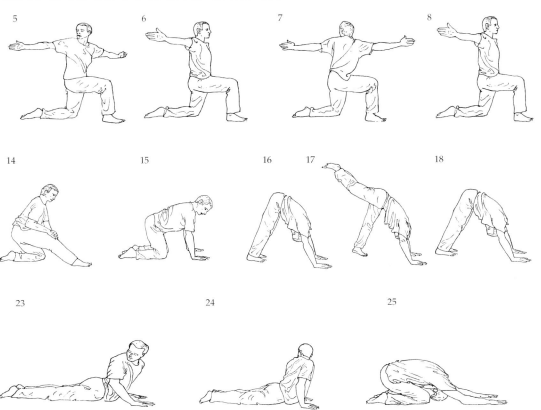

5   6   7   8

14   15   16   17   18

23   24   25

POLAIR GUIDES

—going to the heart of it!

DON'T HOLD YOUR BREATH · Jenny Beeken
None of us breathes as well as we might! This is a book about improving health through simple, easily-acquired techniques of breathing better. Illustrated by Janita Stenhouse. ISBN 0-9545389-9-4

IF I CHANGE, SO CAN THE WORLD · Paula Pluck
Forty positive steps to global togetherness based on the principle that what I do in my own little world permeates out into the whole consciousness. ISBN 1-905398-06-9

INCENSE · Jennie Harding
Create your own special blends of incense to use around the home. ISBN 0-9545389-7-8

MAKING COMPLEMENTARY THERAPIES WORK FOR YOU · Gaye Mack
A book designed to make the choice of complementary therapy simple, the therapy relationship better, and the results deeper and more lasting. ISBN 1-905398--07-7

WHY MEDITATION WORKS · James Baltzell
A doctor writes in confirmation of the widespread belief that meditation has enormous potential for aiding recovery, improving immunity, relieving stress, reducing sclerosis—and a whole lot more! With instructions for beginning meditation and developing a regular meditation practice. ISBN 1-905398-08-5

CREATIVITY AND YOUR SIX SENSES · Jennie Harding
Behind the five senses is a sixth, intuition. By getting away from the senses' exploitation by advertising and back into touch with their immediate effects on our selves, intuition can be unlocked. ISBN 1-905398-05-0

www.polairpublishing.co.uk